THE COMPLETE DIABETIC COOKBOOK

A Comprehensive Guide To Easy And Mouthwatering Diabetic Scientifically Proven Recipes And Ideas For Low-Carb Breads, Cakes, Cookies And More To Reverse Diabetes Without Drugs

Kristen Vane

The Complete Diabetic Cookbook

The Complete Diabetic Cookbook

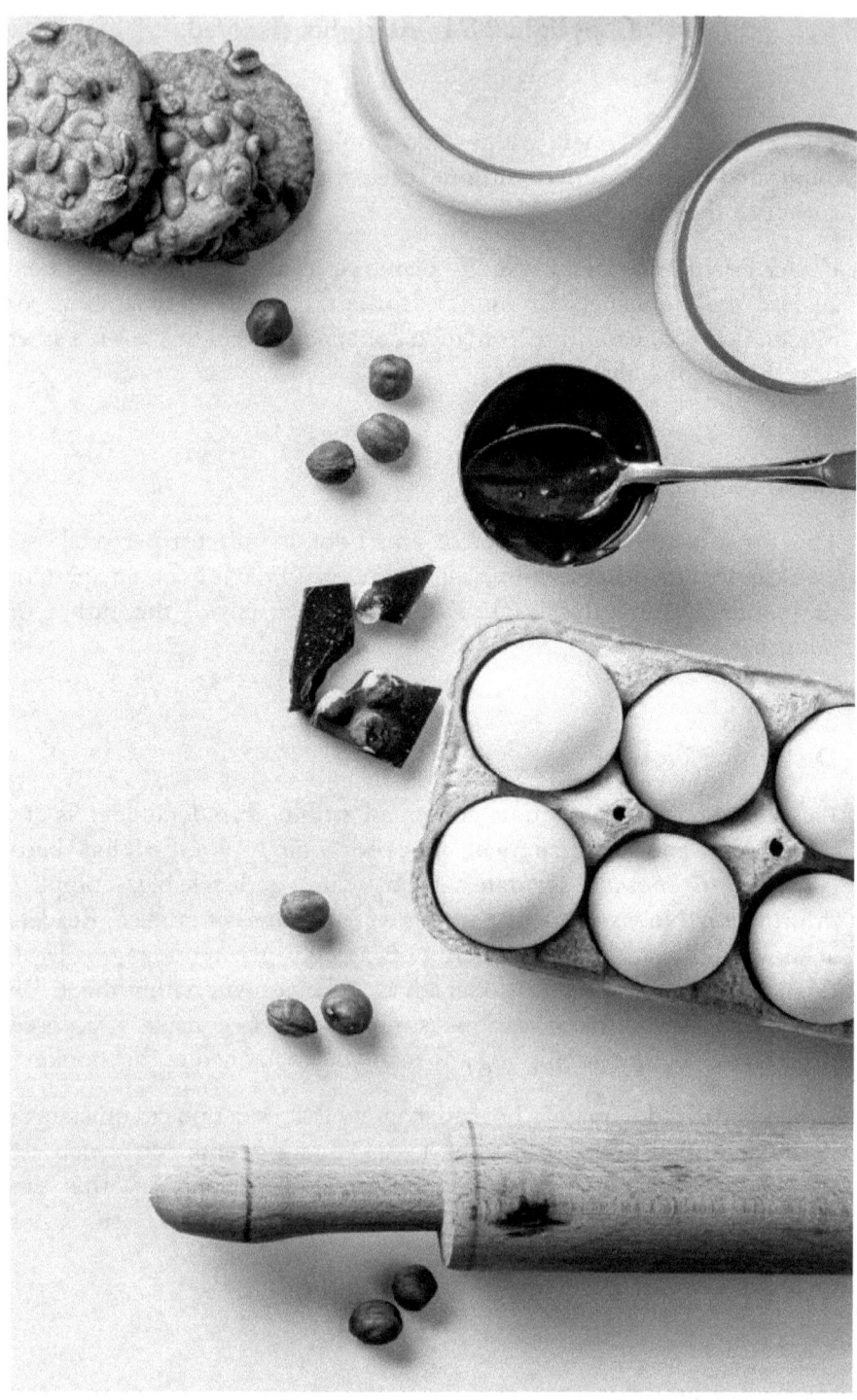

Table of Contents

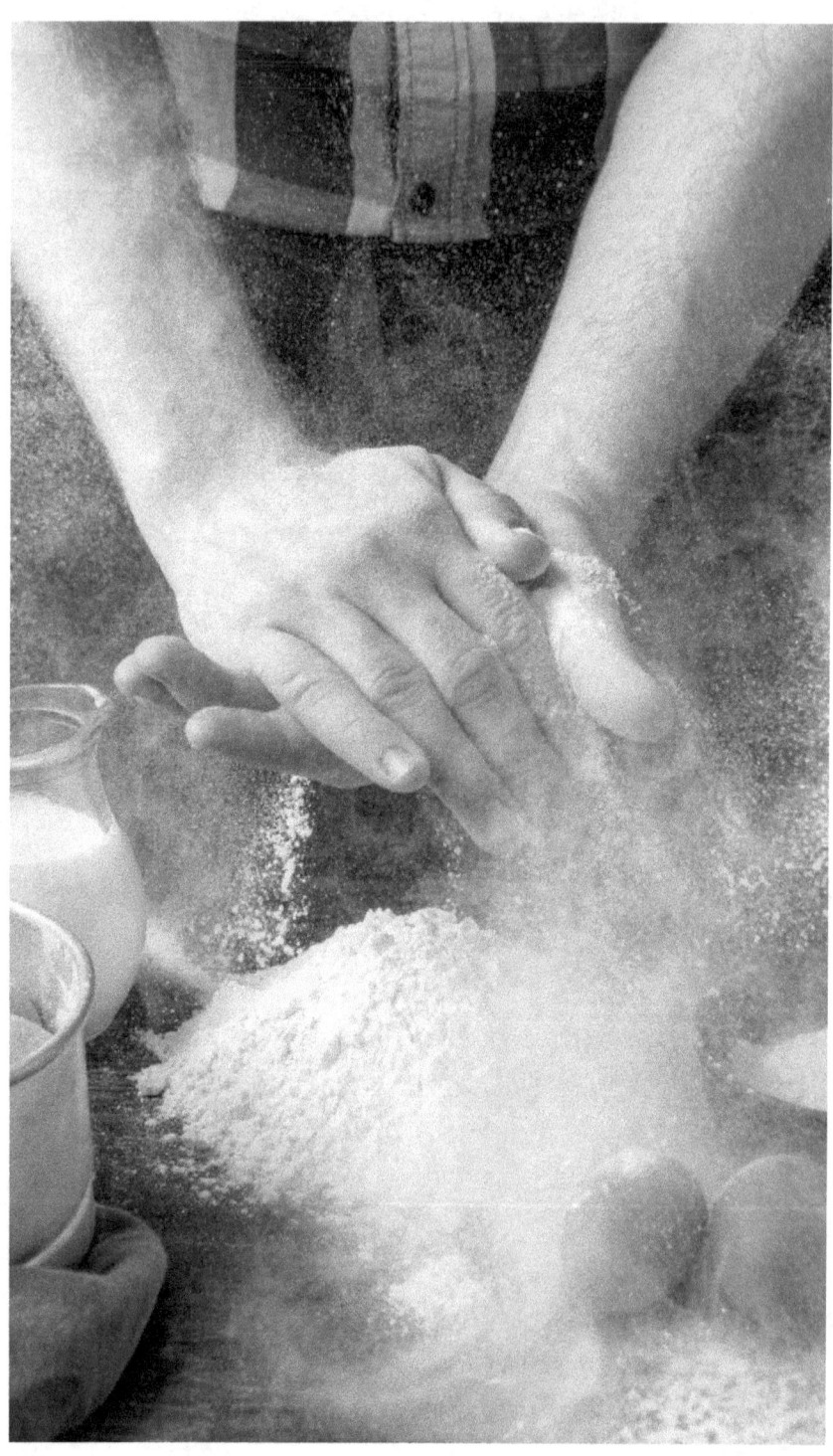

Introduction

Everything you need to know will be reflected in this book; you don't have to go shopping for ingredients. Some recipes call for a little creativity to get everything right, but this is not too much to ask. It is a trivial price to recompense for a great-tasting meal without all the sugar and other sweeteners.

Diabetic Dessert Cookbook provides you with many different recipes, from simple muffins to fantastic cakes. Some of the recipes in this book are very simple to make, while others require more time and effort.

Even if you are a diabetic, you still can enjoy different filling beverages that are low in carbohydrates, refined sugar, and preservatives. The next step is to tick on your favorite recipes and head to the nearest supermarket to purchase the ingredients. Always remember to buy them fresh!

Diabetic foods are the perfect solution to enjoy healthy foods at home every day. Recipes prepared according to these guidelines take care of not only your health but also your cravings to enjoy delicious foods. They greatly assist in keeping your weight under check.

Life with diabetes should not be hard. It is not the end—it is the beginning. With healthy dietary management, you can lead a life free from the negative effects of high (or low) blood sugar levels.

Cook your way to well-being and liveliness with these recipes and tips. Good things are made for sharing, so please help a friend find out about this way of life. Call them over for a meal, talk about diabetes, and let's help create awareness as we feast on every delectable spoonful of diabetic cooking made easy.

Hence, eating healthy food, being physically active will keep your glucose level in check and make sure your body does not become overweight or obese. The most significant thing you can do is make sure the quality of your lifestyle is healthy, which majorly consists of you being conscious of what you eat and how much you are willing to follow the rules. There are many ways to live a healthy life, including keep track of your sugar level. Lower your diabetes chances, make sure your glucose level is under control, or not experience pre-diabetic symptoms. But, if you already have developed diabetes, you need to increase the effort to live a healthy, balanced life.

Chapter 1.

Diabetic Bread Recipes

1. Flaxseed Bread

Preparation Time: 9 Minutes

Cooking Time: 30 Minutes

Servings: 6

Ingredients: color

- 1 teaspoon of salt

- 1/3 cup of olive oil

- 2 cups of flaxseed meal

- ½ cup of water

- 1 tablespoon of baking powder

- 2 tablespoons of maple syrup

- 4 to 5 Beaten pasteurized eggs

Directions:

1. Preheat the oven to around 350°F.

2. Line a 10* 15-inch baking tray with parchment paper.

3. Whisk together your dry ingredients, then add them to the wet ingredients and combine the mixture very well.

4. Set the batter aside for around 3 minutes until it thickens up.

5. Pour your batter into your already prepared tray and spread it into the bottom, but make sure to keep it away from the sides of the pan.

6. Spread the batter into the shape of a rectangle for about 1 inch or two from the end of the pan.

7. Place the baking pan in the oven and bake it for around 30 minutes.

8. Once the bread gets brown, remove it from the oven and set it aside to cool down for around 5 minutes.

9. Slice the bread, then serve and enjoy it!

Nutrition:

- Calories: 187

- Fat: 11g

- Carbohydrates: 7g

- Protein: 8g

2. Gluten-Free Garlic Bread

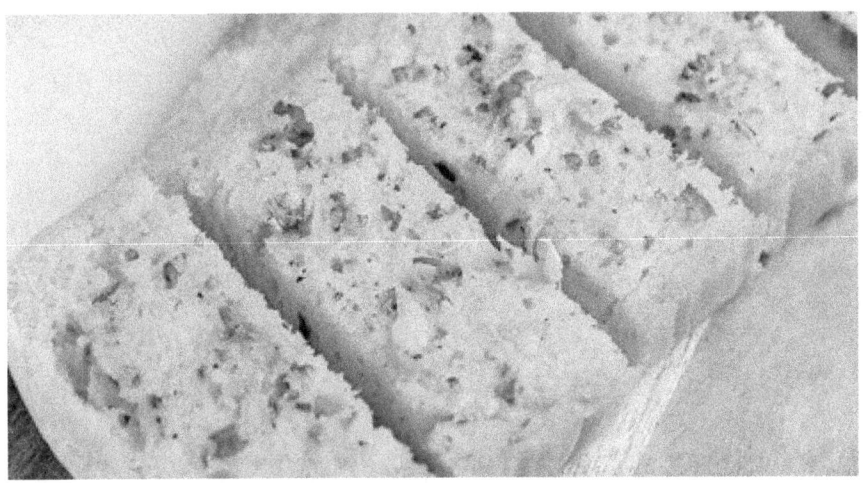

Preparation Time: 9 Minutes

Cooking Time: 40 Minutes

Servings: 5

Ingredients:

- 2 egg whites

- 1 and ¼ cups of boiling water

- 2 teaspoons of apple cider vinegar

- 1 teaspoon of sea salt

- 2 teaspoons of baking powder

- 5 tablespoons of ground Psyllium husk powder

- 1 and ¼ cups of almond flour

For the Garlic butter:

- ½ teaspoon of salt

- 1 Minced garlic clove

- 4 oz of butter

- 2 tablespoons of finely chopped parsley

Directions:

1. Preheat your oven to around 360°F, and then combine your dry ingredients into a deep and large mixing bowl.

2. Pour the boiling water; then add the egg whites and the vinegar to the bowl and keep whisking for around 1 minute, but make sure to not over mix.

3. With moist hands, form around ten pieces.

4. Roll the ten pieces into buns and then place them over a baking sheet.

5. Bake your buns for around 40 minutes in the oven. Meanwhile, prepare the garlic butter by mixing its ingredients and then refrigerate it.

6. Once your buns are ready, set them aside to cool for around 10 minutes.

7. Cut the buns into halves and then spread the butter on every half.

8. Raise the heat to around 425°F, and then bake it for about 15 minutes.

9. Serve and enjoy!

Nutrition:

- Calories: 180

- Fat: 9g

- Carbohydrates: 12g

- Protein: 5g

3. Cloud Bread

Preparation Time: 10 Minutes

Cooking Time: 15 Minutes

Servings: 10

Ingredients:

- 4 eggs, large & separated

- ½ teaspoon Garlic Powder

- ½ teaspoon Cream of Tartar

- ½ teaspoon Sea Salt

- 2 oz. Cream Cheese, low-fat

- 1 teaspoon Italian Seasoning

Directions:

1. Preheat the oven to 300°F.

2. Next, keep the egg whites in a large mixing bowl, and spoon in the cream of tartar.

3. Whip it on high power until it turns to soft meringue peaks. Transfer to another bowl.

4. Place the cream cheese into the large bowl and whip on high power to soften.

5. Stir in the eggs one by one into the mixture and whisk them well each time before adding each egg. Repeat the procedure until the whole mixture becomes smooth.

6. Spoon in the Italian seasoning, salt, and garlic powder.

7. Gently fold the egg whites into the mixture while maintaining the foamy texture.

8. Take ¼ cup portion of the mixture to the greased baking sheet and spread to 4-inch circles. Leave ample space between each.

9. Finally, bake them for 15 to 20 minutes or until they get golden on the outside and firm inside.

10. Let them cool, and then serve.

11. Tip: You can reduce the amount of garlic powder if desired.

Nutrition:

- Calories: 36

- Carbohydrates: 1g

- Protein: 2g

- Fat: 2g

Chapter 2.

Diabetic Snacks and Treats

Recipes

4. Chocolate Chip Blondies

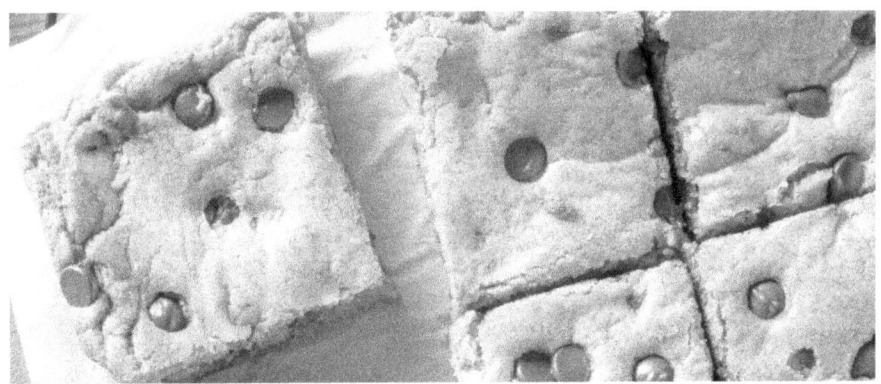

Preparation Time: 6 Minutes

Cooking Time: 21 Minutes

Servings: 12

Ingredients:

- 1 egg

- ½ cup semisweet chocolate chips

- 1/3 cup flour

- 1/3 cup whole wheat flour

- ¼ cup Splenda brown sugar

- ¼ cup sunflower oil

- 2 tablespoons honey

- 1 teaspoon vanilla

- ½ teaspoon baking powder

- ¼ teaspoon salt

- Non-stick cooking spray

Directions:

1. Heat the oven to 350°F. Spray an 8-inch square baking dish with cooking spray.

2. In a small bowl, combine the dry ingredients.

3. In a large bowl, whisk together egg, oil, honey, and vanilla. Stir in the dry ingredients just until combined. Stir in chocolate chips.

4. Spread the batter in the prepared dish. Bake 20-22 minutes or until they pass the toothpick test. Cool on a wire rack, then cut into bars.

Nutrition:

- Calories: 136

- Protein: 2g

- Fat: 6g

5. Cinnamon Apple Chips

Preparation Time: 6 Minutes

Cooking Time: 11 Minutes

Servings: 2

Ingredients:

- 1 medium apple, thinly sliced

- ¼ teaspoon cinnamon

- ¼ teaspoon nutmeg

- Non-stick cooking spray

Directions:

1. Heat the oven to 375°F. Spray a baking sheet with cooking spray.

2. Place apples in a mixing bowl and add spices. Toss to coat.

3. Arrange the apples, in a single layer, on the prepared pan. Bake 4 minutes, turn apples over, and bake four more minutes.

4.   Serve immediately or store in an air-tight container.

Nutrition:

- Calories: 58

- Protein: 0.1g

- Fat: 0.3g

6. Cinnamon Apple Popcorn

Preparation Time: 31 Minutes

Cooking Time: 50 Minutes

Servings: 11

Ingredients:

- 4 tablespoon margarine, melted

- 10 cups plain popcorn

- 2 cups dried apple rings, unsweetened and chopped

- ½ cup walnuts, chopped

- 2 tablespoons Splenda brown sugar

- 1 teaspoon cinnamon

- ½ teaspoon vanilla

Directions:

1. Heat the oven to 250 degrees.

2. Place chopped apples in a 9x13-inch baking dish and bake for 20 minutes. Remove from the oven and stir in popcorn and nuts.

3. In a small bowl, whisk together margarine, vanilla, Splenda, and cinnamon. Drizzle evenly over popcorn and toss to coat.

4. Bake 30 minutes, stirring quickly every 10 minutes. If apples start to turn dark brown, remove them immediately.

5. Pout onto waxed paper to cool for at least 30 minutes. Store in an air-tight container.

Nutrition:

- Calories: 133

- Protein: 3g

- Fat: 8g

7. Crab & Spinach Dip

Preparation Time: 9 Minutes

Cooking Time: 2 Hours

Servings: 10

Ingredients:

- 1 pkg. Frozen chopped spinach, thawed and squeezed nearly dry

- 8 oz. Reduced-fat cream cheese

- 6 ½ oz. Can crabmeat, drained and shredded

- 6 oz. Jar marinated artichoke hearts drained and finely diced

- ¼ teaspoon hot pepper sauce

- Melba toast or whole-grain crackers (optional)

Directions:

1. Remove any shells or cartilage from the crab.

2. Place all ingredients in a small crockpot. Cover and cook on high 1 ½ - 2 hours, or until heated through and cream cheese is melted. Stir after 1 hour.

3. Serve with Melba toast or whole-grain crackers. The serving size is ¼ cup.

Nutrition:

- Calories: 106

- Protein: 5g

- Fat: 8g

The Complete Diabetic Cookbook

Chapter 3.

Diabetic Bars Recipes

8. Sugar Cookie Bars

Preparation Time: 11 Minutes

Cooking Time: 18 Minutes

Servings: 16

Ingredients:

For the Bars:

- 2 tablespoons of Coconut flour

- 200g (2 cups) blanched Almond flour

- ½ cup of granulated Erythritol-based Sweetener

- ½ teaspoon of baking powder

- ½ teaspoon of Vanilla extract

- 1 large egg

- ¼ teaspoon of salt

- 1 Stick (½ cup) unsalted butter, melted

For the Vanilla Frosting:

- ¼ cup (2 oz.) of softened Cream Cheese

- ½ cup (1 stick) of unsalted butter

- ½ cup powdered Erythritol-based Sweetener

- 2-4 tablespoon of heavy Whipping Cream kept at room temp

- ½ teaspoon of Vanilla extract

- 1 tablespoon of Coconut Sprinkles

Directions:

Bars:

1. Heat the oven to 325°F and grease a nine-inch baking pan.

2. Whisk the baking powder, salt, sweetener, vanilla extract, egg, and butter in a large bowl until it is well mixed.

3. Evenly spread the dough in the greased baking pan and bake for 18 minutes until the sides appear golden brown. At this point, the middle will remain soft. Take out of the oven and allow to completely cool in the pan.

Assemble and Frosting:

4. Beat in cream cheese and butter using an electric mixer in a medium bowl until smooth. Add the powdered sweetener and beat.

5. Add one tablespoon of the heavy cream until frosting becomes spreadable. Beat in the vanilla extract until well incorporated.

6. Evenly spread frosting on the top of the cookie and make sure to garnish with coconut sprinkles. Slice into 16 bars.

Nutrition:

- Fat: 20.5g

- Carbs: 3.9g

- Protein: 3.9g

- Calories: 218

9. Dairy-Free Peanut Butter Bars

Preparation Time: 18 Minutes

Cooking Time: 5 Minutes

Servings: 16

Bar

- 2 tablespoons plus ½ cup of coconut oil

- ¾ cup of salted Creamy Peanut Butter

- 2/3 cup of powdered Erythritol-based Sweetener

- 1 teaspoon Vanilla extract

- 200g (2 cups) of defatted Peanut flour

Chocolate Glaze

- 3 oz. of sugarless dark chopped Chocolate

- 1 tablespoon of Coconut oil

Directions:

Preparing the Bars:

1. Line a 9-inch baking pan using parchment paper.

2. Mix the coconut oil and peanut butter in a large bowl. Thoroughly whisk the mixture until smooth. Stir in vanilla extract and sweetener until it becomes thoroughly mixed.

3. Add the peanut flour and stir so that the dough sticks close. Firmly press the dough and evenly flatten it on a coated baking pan. Cover with parchment or wax paper.

Preparing the Assemble and Glaze:

4. Place the coconut oil and the chocolate in a microwaveable bowl. In 30-second increments, microwave on high power until smooth and melted.

5. Pour the glaze on the top of the bars, and with a knife, spread it to the sides. Refrigerate for about an hour so that the chocolate becomes set.

6. Cut into sixteen bars.

Nutrition:

- Fat: 19g

- Carbs: 7.2g

- Protein: 5.5g

- Calories: 211

The Complete Diabetic Cookbook

Chapter 4.

Diabetic Tarts and Crumbles Recipes

10.Sugar-Free Pear Pie

Preparation Time: 9 Minutes

Cooking Time: 60 Minutes

Servings: 8

Ingredients:

For the Crust:

- 1 cup all-purpose flour

- 1/4 cup ground walnuts

- 1 Pinch salt

- 1/4 cup butter, chilled and cubed

- 2-4 tablespoons cold water

For the Filling:

- 4 Ripe pears, peeled, cored, and sliced

- 2 eggs

- 1 cup heavy cream

- 1 teaspoon vanilla extract

- 1 teaspoon cornstarch

Directions:

1. Preheat your oven to 350°F and prepare a round pie pan.

2. To make the crust, mix all the ingredients in a food processor and pulse until well combined.

3. Transfer the dough to a floured working surface and roll it into a thin sheet.

4. Transfer the dough into your prepared pan and press it well on the bottom and sides. Trim the edges if needed.

5. For the filling, arrange the pear slices into the crust.

6. In a bowl, mix the cream, vanilla, eggs, and cornstarch and pour this mixture over the pears.

7. Bake in the oven for 40 minutes or until golden brown and set.

8. Allow the pie to cool completely before slicing and serving.

Nutrition:

- Calories: 121

- Total Carbs: 12g

- Fat: 3g

- Protein: 14g

11. Peanut Butter Smooth Pie

Preparation Time: 7 Minutes

Cooking Time: 60 Minutes

Servings: 9

Ingredients:

For the Crust:

- 1 1/2 cups sugar-free cookie crumbs

- 4 tablespoons butter, melted

- 1 tablespoon peanut butter

For the Filling:

- 8 oz. Low fat cream cheese

- 1 cup smooth peanut butter

- 4 drops stevia extract

- 1 teaspoon vanilla extract

- 1 1/2 cups heavy cream, whipped

Directions:

1. Preheat your oven to 350°F and prepare a round pie pan.

2. For the crust, mix the ingredients in a food processor and pulse until well combined.

3. Transfer the mixture into your pie pan and press it well on the bottom and sides of the pan.

4. Bake the crust in the oven for 10-15 minutes or until golden brown. Remove from the oven when done and let it cool completely.

5. For the filling, mix the cream cheese with peanut butter, stevia and vanilla until smooth.

6. Fold in the whipped heavy cream, then spoon the filling into the pie crust.

7. Refrigerate until serving.

Nutrition:

- Calories: 127

- Total Carbs: 14g

- Fat: 3g

- Protein: 19g

12.Raspberry Almond Tart

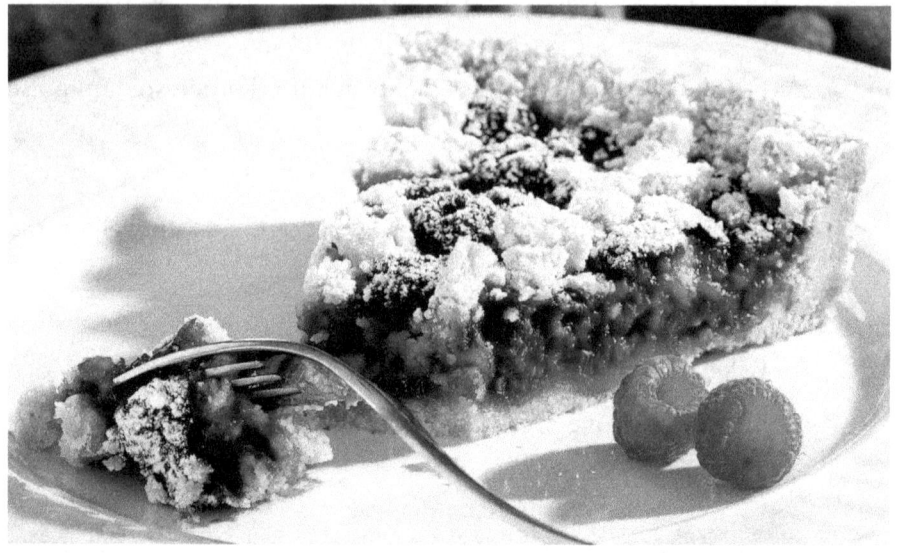

Preparation Time: 10 Minutes

Cooking Time: 30 Minutes

Servings: 4

Ingredients:

- 5 egg whites

- 1 teaspoon vanilla

- 1 1/2 cups raspberries

- 1 Lemon zest, grated

- 1 cup almond flour

- 1/2 cup Swerve

- 1/2 cup butter, melted

- 1 teaspoon baking powder

Directions:

1. Preheat the oven to 375°F/190°C.

2. Grease a tart tin with cooking spray and set it aside.

3. In a large bowl, whisk egg whites until foamy.

4. Add the sweetener, baking powder, vanilla, lemon zest, and almond flour and mix until well combined.

5. Add melted butter and stir well.

6. Pour the batter into the tart tin and top with raspberries.

7. Bake in preheated oven for 20-23 minutes. Serve and enjoy.

Nutrition:

- Calories: 378

- Fat: 8g

- Carbohydrates 14g

- Protein: 11g

Chapter 5.

Diabetic Muffins Recipes

13.Sugar-Free Blueberry Muffins

Preparation Time: 9 Minutes

Cooking Time: 28 Minutes

Servings: 6

Ingredients:

- Vegetable oil cooking spray

- 2 tablespoons wheat (or oat) bran and one tablespoon soy flour, mixed together

- 1 cup soy flour

- 1/2 cup sugar substitute

- 1 teaspoon baking powder

- 2 eggs

- 1/2 cup heavy cream

- 1/3 cup club soda

- 1/2 cup blueberries

Directions:

1. Preheat the oven to 375°F.

2. Spray a 6-cup muffin tin with vegetable oil cooking spray.

3. Evenly sprinkle the pan with the wheat bran and soy flour mix, being careful to coat the sides of the cups also; this will prevent sticking.

4. In a bowl using a wire whisk, mix all the remaining ingredients, except the blueberries, until well blended.

5. Fold in the blueberries and fill the six muffin cups evenly with the batter.

6. Place on the center rack of the oven and bake for 20 to 25 minutes, or until the tops turn golden brown and a toothpick stuck in the center comes out clean.

7. Take out from the oven and let cool.

8. Serve and enjoy!

Nutrition:

- Calories: 125

- Total Carbs: 14g

- Fat: 5g

- Protein: 19g

14. No Sugar Sweet Potato Muffins

Preparation Time: 11 Minutes

Cooking Time: 30 Minutes

Servings: 6

Ingredients:

- 3/4 cup almond meal

- 1 teaspoon baking soda

- 1/4 teaspoon salt

- 1 teaspoon ground cinnamon

- 1/2 teaspoon ground cardamom

- 1/4 teaspoon ground cloves

- 1/4 teaspoon anise powder

- 2/3 cup coconut cream

- 3 tablespoons almond butter

- 4 large eggs, at room temperature

- Zest of 1 orange

- 2 tablespoons vanilla extract

- 1 tablespoon apple cider vinegar

- 1 cup raw grated sweet potato

- 1/2 cup sugar substitute

Directions:

1. Preheat the oven to 350°F.

2. Line a muffin tin with muffin liners.

3. In a medium bowl, mix almond meal, baking soda, salt, and spices. Mix well.

4. Add the coconut butter and almond butter and mix well again.

5. Add the eggs, zest, vanilla, vinegar, sweet potato, and sweetener.

6. Mix until smooth.

7. Sweeten to taste.

8. Fill muffin cups about 3/4 full with batter.

9. Bake 22-28 minutes, or until a wooden toothpick comes out clean.

Nutrition:

- Calories: 117

- Total Carbs: 12g

- Fat: 3g

- Protein: 11g

15.Sugar-Free English Muffins

Preparation Time: 11 Minutes

Cooking Time: 28 Minutes

Servings: 6

Ingredients:

- 1 egg

- 1 tablespoon coconut flour

- 1 teaspoon psyllium husk powder

- 1 tablespoon water

- Pinch of baking powder

- Pinch of salt

Directions:

1. Whisk together the egg, olive oil, and water in a mug or a small microwavable bowl or ramekin

2. Add the coconut flour, psyllium husk, baking powder, and salt, and whisk until there are no lumps

3. Microwave on high for about 1 ½-2 minutes until it is cooked through.

4. Serve and enjoy!

Nutrition:

- Calories: 124

- Total Carbs: 12g

- Fat: 8g

- Protein: 19g

Chapter 6.

Diabetic Cookies Recipes

16.Banana Cookies

Preparation Time: 9 Minutes

Cooking Time: 30 Minutes

Servings: 12

Ingredients:

- 2 1/4 cups flour

- 1 teaspoon baking soda

- 1 teaspoon salt

- 3/4 cup unsweetened applesauce

- 2 egg whites

- 1/2 cup Splenda sugar substitute

- 1/4 cup sugar

- 1/2 cup Splenda brown sugar blend

- 1 medium banana, mashed

- 1 teaspoon vanilla

- 1 1/4 cups semi-sweet chocolate chips

- 4 Marshmallows, shredded

Directions:

1. Preheat the oven to 350°F.

2. Stir flour, salt, and baking soda in a bowl, then set aside. Beat applesauce, egg whites, and sugars with a mixer. Mix in bananas and vanilla.

3. Slowly add flour mixture to the mixer. Add chocolate chips and marshmallows. Drop by spoonfuls on the cookie sheet.

4. Bake for 15 minutes.

Nutrition:

- Calories: 83

- Fat: 2g

- Carbohydrates: 16g

- Protein: 1g

17. Raisin Oatmeal Cookies

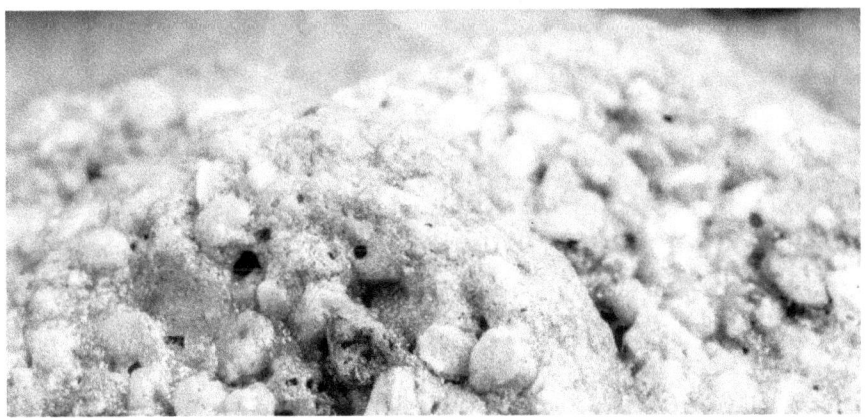

Preparation Time: 11 Minutes

Cooking Time: 30 Minutes

Servings: 6

Ingredients:

- 1 cup self-rising flour

- 1/2 cup butter

- 2 tablespoons white Splenda granular

- 2 tablespoons milk

- 1 1/2 cups quick oats

- 1 egg

- 1/4 teaspoon cinnamon

- 1/3 cup Splenda brown sugar blend

- 1/2 teaspoon vanilla

- 1/2 cup dark raisins

Directions:

1. Preheat the oven to 325 degrees.

2. In a bowl, mix the flour with the cinnamon.

3. In a separate bowl, cream the butter and both of the sugars until fluffy. Add the egg, milk, and vanilla. Gradually add the flour mixture.

4. Stir in oats and raisins.

5. Drop by teaspoonfuls if you desire small cookies or tablespoons if you desire larger cookies onto parchment paper.

6. Bake until golden brown, 10-12 minutes. Cool on wire racks.

Nutrition:

- Calories: 95

- Fat: 4.5g

- Carbohydrates: 12g

- Protein: 2g

18.Chocolate Cookies

Preparation Time: 11 Minutes

Cooking Time: 25 Minutes

Servings: 6

Ingredients:

- 1 cup all-purpose flour

- 1/4 teaspoon baking soda

- 1/4 cup light margarine

- 1/2 cup granulated Splenda

- 1/3 cup unsweetened cocoa powder

- 1/4 cup packed Splenda brown sugar blend

- 1/4 cup buttermilk

- 1 teaspoon vanilla extract

- 1 tablespoon confectioner's sugar

Directions:

1. In a small bowl, combine flour and baking soda; set aside.

2. In a medium saucepan, melt margarine; remove from the heat. Stir in granulated Splenda, cocoa powder, and Splenda brown sugar blend. Stir in buttermilk and vanilla. Stir in flour mixture just until combined.

3. Cover and chill dough for 1 hour; the dough should be stiff.

4. Preheat the oven to 350°F. Lightly coat two baking sheets with cooking spray.

5. Drop the dough by rounded teaspoons onto baking sheets.

6. Bake 8 to 10 minutes, or until edges are set. Cool 1 minute, then transfer to a wire rack to cool completely.

7. Sprinkle with confectioner's sugar.

Nutrition:

- Calories: 66

- Fat: 2g

- Carbohydrates: 12g

- Protein: 1g

19.Cheesecake Cookies

Preparation Time: 13 Minutes

Cooking Time: 25 Minutes

Servings: 6

Ingredients:

- 1/2 cup graham cracker crumbs, low fat

- 3 cup oats, rolled,

- 1 1/2 cup Splenda

- 1/2 cup unsweetened cocoa powder

- 1/2 cup fat-free milk

- 1/2 cup margarine

- 1/2 cup reduced-fat peanut butter

- 1/2 teaspoon orange zest

- 1/2 teaspoon vanilla extract

- 6 tablespoon light cream cheese

- 1 tablespoon unsweetened pineapple juice

Directions:

1. Crush graham crackers, then in a large saucepan, stir in the Splenda, cocoa, milk, and margarine over medium heat until dissolved.

2. Bring the mix to a boil. Make sure the oatmeal is cooked.

3. Remove from the heat, and stir in the peanut butter and vanilla until well mixed.

4. Blend in the oatmeal and graham crumbs. By teaspoon, drop onto waxed paper. Refrigerate or store in another cool place until firm.

For the frosting:

5. Combine the cream cheese, vanilla, zest, juice, and frost cookies.

Nutrition:

- Calories: 86

- Fat: 5g

- Carbohydrates: 11g

- Protein: 3g

Chapter 7.

Diabetic Custard Recipes

20. Get Well Custard

Preparation Time: 14 Minutes

Cooking Time: 55 Minutes

Servings: 10

Ingredients:

- 4 large eggs

- 1/2 cup sugar

- 1/4 teaspoon salt

- 1 teaspoon vanilla extract

- 4 cups whole milk

- Ground nutmeg

Directions:

1. Lightly beat eggs in a bowl; whisk in vanilla, salt, and sugar. Warm milk; add to the egg mixture slowly. Put through a strainer into one 1/2-qt round baking dish, then sprinkle nutmeg.

2. Put the baking dish in a bigger pan; put 1-inch hot water in a bigger pan. Bake at 350°F till a knife inserted in the middle comes out clean for 55-60 minutes. Even after chilling, it'll jiggle and be very soft. Cool to room temperature; chill till serving.

Nutrition:

- Calories: 129

- Protein: 6g

- Fat: 5g

- Carbohydrate: 15g

21.Macadamia Crusted Custards

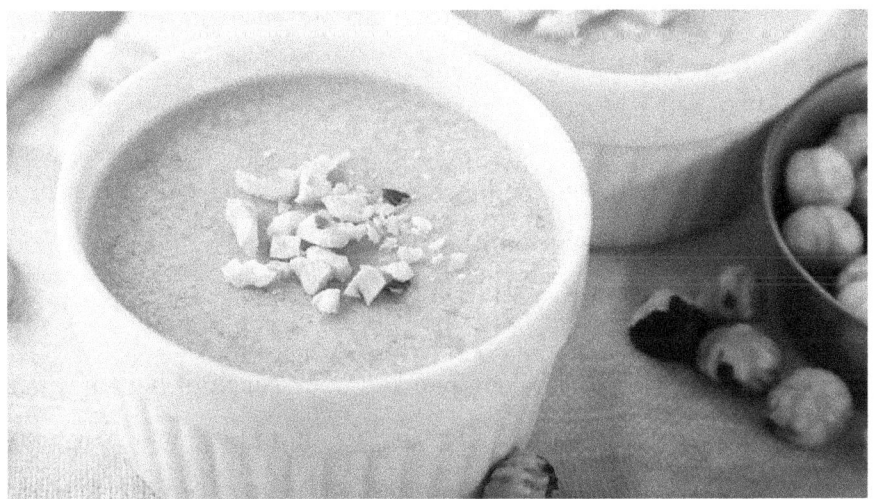

Preparation Time: 9 Minutes

Cooking Time: 25 Minutes

Servings: 2

Ingredients:

- 2 large egg yolks

- 1 large egg

- 3/4 cup half-and-half cream

- 4-1/2 teaspoons sugar

- 1/2 teaspoon rum extract

- 1/8 teaspoon salt

- 1/4 cup finely chopped macadamia nuts, walnuts, or pecans

Directions:

1. Whisk cream, egg, and egg yolks, sugar, salt, and extract in a small mixing bowl until incorporated. Pour mixture into two ungreased 6-oz custard cups. Scatter with nuts.

2. Arrange cups in a baking pan and pour 1 inch of boiling water into the pan. Uncover and bake for 25 to 30 minutes at 350° until a knife comes out clean from the center. Take the pan out of the oven and place it onto a wire rack to cool for 15 minutes. Chill in the refrigerator.

Nutrition:

- Calories: 368

- Protein: 10g

- Fat: 28g

- Carbohydrate: 15g

22. Mini Pumpkin Custards

Preparation Time: 25 Minutes

Cooking Time: 20 Minutes

Servings: 8

Ingredients:

- 1/2 cup half-and-half cream

- 1/2 cup heavy whipping cream

- 3 large egg yolks

- 2 tablespoons plus 2 teaspoons sugar

- 1/8 teaspoon ground cinnamon

- A dash of salt, ground cloves, and nutmeg

- 1/3 cup canned pumpkin

- 1/4 cup maple syrup

- 1/2 teaspoon vanilla extract

- Whipped cream and additional ground nutmeg

Directions:

1. Heat the heavy cream and half and half in a small saucepan till bubbles form around the pan's sides. Whisk nutmeg, cloves, and salt, cinnamon, sugar, and egg yolks in a small bowl.

2. Take the cream off the heat; mix the small hot cream amount into the egg mixture. Put all back into the pan, constantly mixing; mix in vanilla, syrup, and pumpkin.

3. Put into 8 2-oz. ramekins/stoneware demitasse cups. Put cups in baking pan; to the pan, add 1-in. boiling water.

4. Bake at 325°F, uncovered, till centers just set (it'll jiggle) for 20-25 minutes for the ramekins, 25-30 minutes for the demitasse cups. Take the cups from the water bath and cool for 10 minutes, then cover; refrigerate for a minimum of 4 hours. Garnish with extra nutmeg and whipped cream.

Nutrition:

- Calories: 138

- Protein: 2g

- Fat: 9g

- Carbohydrate: 13g

23.Pumpkin Pecan Custard

Preparation Time: 20 Minutes

Cooking Time: 35 Minutes

Servings: 6

Ingredients:

For the Custard:

- 3 eggs

- 2/3 cup lightly packed brown sugar

- 1/2 teaspoon ground cinnamon

- 1/2 teaspoon vanilla extract

- 1/4 teaspoon ground allspice

- 1/4 teaspoon ground ginger

- 1/4 teaspoon ground nutmeg

- 1/4 teaspoon ground cloves

- 1 1/2 cups canned pumpkin puree

- 1 cup low-fat evaporated milk

For the Topping:

- 2 tablespoons brown sugar

- 1 tablespoon all-purpose flour

- 1/4 teaspoon ground cinnamon

- 1/2 tablespoons melted butter

- 3 tablespoons chopped toasted pecans

For the Garnish:

- Whipped cream (optional)

Directions:

1. Preheat the oven to 180°C/350°F. Grease 6 180-ml/6-oz ramekins lightly; put onto a baking sheet.

2. Lightly beat eggs with a fork in a medium bowl/big glass measuring cup. Add cloves, nutmeg, ginger, allspice, vanilla, cinnamon, and 150-ml/2/3 cup brown sugar; mix in pumpkin puree till blended. Mix the evaporated milk slowly; put it evenly in the prepped ramekins.

3. Bake for 20 minutes.

4. Meanwhile, for topping, mix 1-ml/1/4 teaspoon cinnamon, flour, and 30-ml/2 tablespoons brown sugar in a small bowl. Add melted butter; mix in pecans.

5. Remove from the oven after baking the custards for 20 minutes; sprinkle the nut mixture evenly on the custards. Bake till an inserted knife near the middle comes out clean for 15 minutes.

6. Put onto a rack; cool. Serve chilled/warm, with, if desired, a dollop of whipped cream.

Nutrition:

*   Calories: 250

*   Fat: 7.4g

*   Carbohydrate: 4.5g

*   Protein: 7.6g

Chapter 8.

Diabetic Desserts Recipes

Generic Desserts Recipes

24. Cream Cheese Swirl Brownies

Preparation Time: 10 Minutes

Cooking Time: 20 Minutes

Servings: 12

Ingredients:

- 2 eggs

- ¼ cup unsweetened applesauce

- ¼ cup coconut oil, melted

- 3 tablespoons pure maple syrup, divided

- ¼ cup unsweetened cocoa powder

- ¼ cup coconut flour

- ¼ teaspoon salt

- 1 teaspoon baking powder

- 2 tablespoons low-fat cream cheese

Directions:

1. Preheat the oven to 350°F. Grease an 8-by-8-inch baking dish.

2. In a large mixing bowl, beat the eggs with the applesauce, coconut oil, and 2 tablespoons of maple syrup.

3. Stir in the cocoa powder and coconut flour, and mix well. Sprinkle the salt and baking powder evenly over the surface and mix well to incorporate. Transfer the mixture to the prepared baking dish.

4. In a small, microwave-safe bowl, microwave the cream cheese for 10 to 20 seconds until softened. Add the remaining tablespoon of maple syrup and mix to combine.

5. Drop the cream cheese onto the batter, and use a toothpick or chopstick to swirl it on the surface. Bake for 20 minutes until a toothpick inserted in the center comes out clean. Cool and cut into 12 squares.

6. Store refrigerated in a covered container for up to 5 days.

Nutrition:

- Calories: 84

- Fat: 6g

- Protein: 2g

- Carbohydrates: 6g

25. Greek Yogurt Sundae

Preparation Time: 8 Minutes

Cooking Time: 0 Minutes

Servings: 1

Ingredients:

- ¾ cup plain nonfat Greek yogurt

- ¼ cup mixed berries (blueberries, strawberries, blackberries)

- 2 tablespoons cashew, walnut, or almond pieces

- 1 tablespoon ground flaxseed

- 2 Fresh mint leaves, shredded

Directions:

1. Spoon the yogurt into a small bowl. Top with the berries, nuts, and flaxseed.

2. Garnish with the mint and serve.

Nutrition:

- Calories: 237

- Fat: 11g

- Protein: 21g

- Carbohydrates: 16g

26.Lemon Berry Chiffon

Preparation Time: 14 minutes

Cooking Time: 10 minutes

Servings: 6

Ingredients:

- 1/3 cup fresh lemon juice

- ½ cup sweetener

- 4 large eggs, beaten

- 3 cup fresh berries, such as strawberries, blueberries, and blackberries

Directions:

1. Place lemon juice and sweetener in a small saucepan.

2. Heat gently, stirring until all the sugar has dissolved. Remove from the heat and set aside to cool.

3. Whisk the lemon juice mixture into the eggs and return to the saucepan.

4. Whisk while cooking over low heat until the mixture thickens.

5. After around 5 minutes, the mixture should coat the back of a spoon.

6. Refrigerate for at least an hour.

7. Use the berries to top the lemon chiffon, or you can layer the berries into the serving glasses.

Nutrition:

- Calories: 90

- Total Carbs: 11g

- Fat: 4g

- Protein: 5g

Diabetic Cakes Recipes

27.Angel Food Cake

Preparation Time: 9 Minutes

Cooking Time: 30 Minutes

Servings: 12

Ingredients:

- 1 cup sifted cake flour

- 1 1/2 cups sugar, divided (or sugar substitute equivalent)

- 12 large egg whites

- 1 teaspoon cream of tartar

- 1/4 teaspoon salt

- 1 1/2 teaspoons vanilla extract

- 1 1/2 teaspoons fresh lemon juice

- 1/2 teaspoon almond extract

Directions:

1. Preheat the oven to 325°F.

2. To prepare the cake, lightly spoon flour into a dry measuring cup; level with a knife. Combine flour and 3/4 cup sugar, stirring with a whisk.

3. Place egg whites in a large bowl; beat with a mixer at high speed until foamy. Add cream of tartar and salt; beat until soft peaks form. Add 3/4 cup sugar, two tablespoons at a time, beating until stiff peaks form.

4. Beat in vanilla, juice, and almond extract. Sift 1/4 cup flour mixture over egg white mixture; fold in. Repeat with the remaining flour mixture, 1/4 cup at a time.

5. Spoon the batter into an ungreased 10-inch tube pan, spreading evenly. Break air pockets by cutting through the batter with a knife—Bake at 325°F for 55 minutes or until cake springs back when lightly touched. Invert the pan; cool completely.

6. Loosen cake from the pan sides using a narrow metal spatula. Invert the cake onto a plate.

Nutrition:

- Calories: 146

- Fat: 1g

- Carbs 31g

- Protein: 4g

28.Chocolate Lava Cake

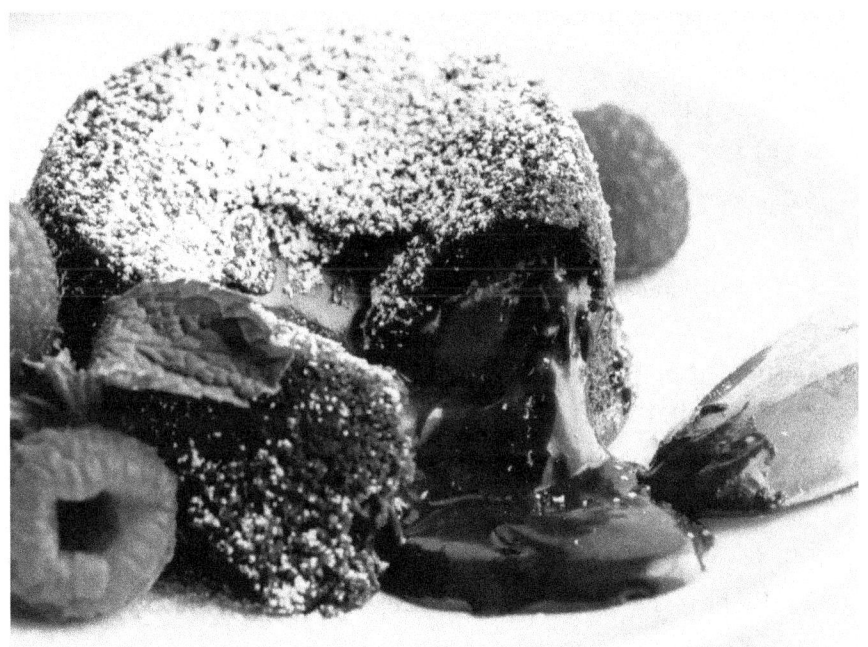

Preparation Time: 7 Minutes

Cooking Time: 13 Minutes

Servings: 8

Ingredients:

- ½ cup raw unsweetened cocoa powder

- ¼ cup butter, melted

- 4 eggs

- ¼ cup sugar-free and gluten-free chocolate sauce

- ½ teaspoon ground cinnamon

- ½ teaspoon sea salt

- 1 teaspoon pure vanilla extract

- ¼ cup raw stevia

Directions:

1. Pour one tablespoon of chocolate sauce into four cavities of an ice cube tray and freeze it.

2. Preheat the oven to 350°F. Prepare four ramekins by greasing with oil or butter.

3. Whisk together the cocoa powder, stevia, cinnamon, and sea salt in a small bowl.

4. Whisk in the eggs, one at a time.

5. Add the melted butter and vanilla extract. Stir until well combined.

6. Fill each prepared ramekin halfway with the mixture.

7. Remove the chocolate sauce from the freezer and place one in each of the ramekins.

8. Cover the chocolate with the remaining cake batter.

9. Bake for 13 to 14 minutes or until just set. Transfer from the oven to a wire rack and allow to cool for 5 minutes.

10. Carefully remove the cakes from the ramekins.

11. Enjoy your tasty and healthy chocolate lava cake by cutting into its molten center.

Nutrition:

- Total Carbohydrates: 6g

- Protein: 8g

- Total Fat: 17g

- Calories: 189

29. Decadent Three-Layered Chocolate Cream Cake

Preparation Time: 30 Minutes

Cooking Time: 60 Minutes

Servings: 8

Ingredients:

- 4 ounces unsweetened chocolate

- ½ cup (1 stick) butter

- 1 ½ cups powdered sweetener, divided

- 3 eggs

- ½ cup + 8 tablespoons raw unsweetened cocoa powder

- 1 Vanilla pod

- Pinch of sea salt

- 1 cup whipping cream

- Coconut whipped cream

- 1 Can of coconut milk, refrigerated overnight

Directions:

1. Preheat the oven to 325°F. Spray a little cooking oil into a pan smaller than 8 inches.

2. Combine the chocolate and butter in a double boiler and melt them together. Stir in ½ cup of sweetener and keep on stirring over low heat until everything is well combined. Remove from the heat and let cool a little bit.

3. Separate the eggs, and beat the whites until stiff peaks form. Add ¼ cup of sweetener little by little.

4. Whisk the yolks together with another ¼ cup of sweetener. Add the chocolate mixture to the yolks and stir well. Mix in ½ cup cocoa, and then scrape the vanilla seeds from the pod and add to the mixture along with salt.

5. Fold in egg whites slowly to the chocolate mixture, but do not over mix.

6. Cook in the preheated oven for 1 hour or until a toothpick comes out clean. Let it cool completely, and then remove it from the pan.

Cream:

7. To prepare the three types of filling, beat the whipping cream for about 6-7 minutes until it gets very thick. Slowly add ½ cup of sweetener.

8. Divide the cream into halves and place one half in a bowl. Divide the remaining cream into halves again and place in the other two separate bowls. You will have three bowls, one with ½ of the cream and two with ¼ of the cream.

9. Take a bowl with ¼ cream, add one tablespoon of cocoa powder and mix well. This will be the lightest-colored cream.

10. Add ½ the cream to the bowl, add three tablespoons of cocoa powder. Mix until well distributed. This will be the middle-colored cream.

11. Add 3–4 tablespoons of cocoa powder to the last bowl with ¼ cream. This will be the darkest cream.

Assembling:

12. Slice the cake horizontally in 3 equal slices using a very sharp knife.

13. Place the bottom part on a serving plate and cover with the middle-colored cream. Repeat with the second layer.

14. Top with the third cake piece and spread the light-colored cream on top, followed by the darkest cream.

15. Cut in 8 slices and enjoy.

Nutrition:

- Total Carbohydrates: 11g

- Protein: 7g

- Total Fat: 27g

- Calories: 304

Chapter 9.

Diabetic Keto Fat Bombs Recipes

30.Fried Fresco Cheese

Preparation Time: 8 Minutes

Cooking Time: 8 Minutes

Servings: 12

Ingredients:

- 2 Pounds Queso fresco

- 2 tablespoons coconut oil

- 1 tablespoon olive oil

- 1 tablespoon chopped basil

Directions:

1. Heat together coconut and olive oil in a pan.

2. Cut the cheese into small cubes.

3. Fry in oil. Make sure to fry all sides until brown.

4. Sprinkle with fresh basil, and enjoy!

Nutrition:

- Calories: 243

- Fat: 19g

- Protein: 16g

- Carbohydrates: 0g

31.Apple Rounds

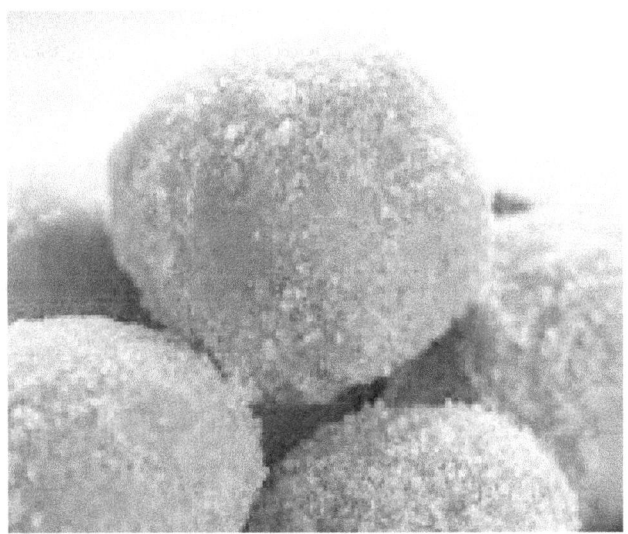

Preparation Time: 3 Hours

Cooking Time: 5 Minutes

Servings: 12

Ingredients:

- 2 Medium-sized apples

- 5 Ounces heavy cream

- ½ cup grass-fed butter

- 2 tablespoons coconut oil

- 1 teaspoon ground cinnamon

- Stevia to taste

- A pinch of salt

Directions:

1. Thinly slice the apples.

2. Melt the coconut oil in a pan and add in the apples and cinnamon. Mix well to coat the apples.

3. Cook until they become tender. Softly mash them with your spoon.

4. Remove from the heat and fold in the rest of the ingredients.

5. Pour into candy molds (preferably apple-shaped) and freeze for about 3 hours.

6. Store in the refrigerator.

Nutrition:

- Calories: 168

- Fat: 12g

- Protein: 0g

- Carbohydrates: 10g

32.Cream Cheese Clouds

Preparation Time: 68 Minutes

Cooking Time: 12 Minutes

Servings: 6

Ingredients:

- ½ cup grass-fed butter

- 8 Ounces cream cheese

- ½ teaspoon vanilla extract

- Stevia to taste

Directions:

1. Whisk everything together using an electric beater until frothy.

2. Drop a spoonful onto a tray and freeze until set.

Nutrition:

- Calories: 134

- Fat: 14g

- Protein: 1g

- Carbohydrates: 1g

Chapter 10.

Diabetic Pudding Recipes

33. Cinnamon Bread Pudding

Preparation Time: 9 Minutes

Cooking Time: 45 Minutes

Servings: 6

Ingredients:

- 4 cups day-old French or Italian bread, cut into ¾-inch cubes

- 2 cups skim milk

- 2 egg whites

- 1 egg

- 4 tablespoons margarine, sliced

- 5 teaspoons Splenda

- 1½ teaspoons cinnamon

- ¼ teaspoon salt

- 1/8 teaspoon ground cloves

Directions:

1. Heat the oven to 350°F (180°C).

2. In a medium saucepan, heat milk and margarine to simmering. Remove from the heat and stir till margarine is completely melted. Let cool for 10 minutes.

3. In a large bowl, beat egg and egg whites until foamy. Add Splenda, spices, and salt. Beat until combined, then add in cooled milk and bread.

4. Transfer the mixture to a 1½ quart baking dish. Place on a roasting pan rack and add 1 inch of hot water to the roaster.

5. Bake until pudding is set and a knife inserted in the center comes out clean, about 40 to 45 minutes.

Nutrition:

- Calories: 363

- Fat: 10.0g

- Protein: 14.0g

- Carbs: 25.1g

Chapter 11.

Diabetic Mousse and Milkshake

Recipes

34.Strawberry Mousse

Preparation Time: 10 Minutes

Cooking Time: 30 Minutes

Servings: 6

Ingredients:

- 1½ cups fresh strawberries, hulled

- 1 2/3 cups chilled unsweetened almond milk

- 2-3 drops liquid stevia

- 1 teaspoon organic vanilla extract

Directions:

1. In a food processor, add all the ingredients and pulse until smooth.

2. Transfer into serving bowls and serve.

3. Meal Prep Tip: Transfer the mousse into an airtight container. Cover the containers and refrigerate for up to 3 days.

Nutrition:

- Calories: 25

- Total Fat: 1.1g

- Total Carbs: 3.4g

- Protein: 0.5g

Chapter 12.

Diabetic Sorbets Recipes

35.Sweet and Sour Watermelon Sorbet

Preparation Time: 19 Minutes

Cooking Time: 0 Minutes

Servings: 6

Ingredients:

- 1 tablespoon lemon juice

- ½ seedless watermelon, frozen and chopped

Directions:

1. Feed the frozen watermelon chunks and lemon juice into the Yonanas Healthy Dessert Maker®.

2. Press down with the plunger.

3. Enjoy.

Nutrition:

- Calories: 114

- Carbohydrates: 4g

- Protein: 3g

- Fat: 15g

36.Mango Sorbet

Preparation Time: 8 Minutes

Cooking Time: 0 Minutes

Servings: 8

Ingredients:

- 4 Mangos, chopped and frozen

- 2 tablespoons lime juice

- 1 cup simple syrup

Directions:

1. Feed 1 cup of frozen mangos into the Yonanas Healthy Dessert Maker® chute.

2. Top with ¼ of the simple syrup and ½ a tablespoon of lime juice.

3. Press down with the plunger.

4. Repeat until all ingredients are used.

5. Enjoy.

Nutrition:

- Calories: 118

- Carbohydrates: 11g

- Protein: 6g

- Fat: 19g

37. Grape Sorbet

Preparation Time: 8 minutes

Cooking Time: 0 minutes

Servings: 2

Ingredients:

- 3 cups frozen green grapes

Directions:

1. Toss grapes into your Yonanas Healthy Frozen Dessert Maker®.

2. Press down with the plunger when the chute gets full.

3. You're done! Enjoy.

Nutrition:

- Calories: 118

- Carbohydrates: 3g

- Protein: 9g

- Fat: 16g

Chapter 13.

Diabetic Fruity Desserts Recipes

38.Figs with Honey & Yogurt

Preparation Time: 5 Minutes

Cooking Time: 10 Minutes

Servings: 4

Ingredients:

- ½ teaspoon vanilla

- 8 oz. Nonfat yogurt

- 2 Figs, sliced

- 1 tablespoon walnuts, chopped and toasted

- 2 teaspoons honey

Directions:

1. Stir the vanilla into yogurt.

2. Mix well.

3. Top with the figs and sprinkle with walnuts.

4. Drizzle with honey and serve.

Nutrition:

-   Calories: 157

-   Carbohydrates: 24g

-   Protein: 7g

Chapter 14.

Diabetic Chocolate Recipes

39.Chocolate Cream-Filled Pumpkin Cupcakes with Vanilla Cream Cheese Frosting

Preparation Time: 8 Minutes

Cooking Time: 45 Minutes

Servings: 6

Ingredients:

- 1 (15-oz.) Can of pure pumpkin

- ½ cup egg whites or two eggs

- 2 eggs

- ½ cup unsweetened applesauce

- ½ cup coconut oil

- 2 oz. Unsweetened baking chocolate

- 1 teaspoon vanilla extract

- 1 teaspoon pure stevia extract

- 2 cups gluten-free flour

- ½ cup unsweetened cocoa powder

- ½ teaspoon salt

- 2 teaspoon baking powder

- 1 teaspoon baking soda

- 2 teaspoon allspice

- 2 teaspoons pumpkin pie spice

- 1 teaspoon xanthan gum

- 1 tablespoon powdered stevia

- Optional: ½ cup chocolate chips

Directions:

1. Preheat the oven to 350°F. Whisk pumpkin, egg whites, eggs, and applesauce together in a bowl. Set aside. Melt coconut oil, chocolate, vanilla, and pure stevia extract in a saucepan over low heat or in a microwavable bowl in 30-second intervals until melted.

2. Whisk flour, cocoa, salt, baking powder, baking soda, spices, xanthan, and powdered stevia together in another bowl. Slowly pour dry ingredients into pumpkin/egg mixture, mixing until combined. Then add melted chocolate mixture and stir to incorporate completely. Stir in optional chocolate chips if using.

3. Pour the batter into a 12-capacity greased muffin tin or use silicone muffin cups. Bake 30 minutes or until the toothpick in the center comes out clean. Allow to cool 5 minutes and then remove from the pan, loosening edges with a butter knife if needed, and finish cooling on a wire rack.

4. Once completely cool, use an apple corer to remove some center of cupcakes. Be careful not to core through the bottom of cupcakes. Make the frosting and use a pastry bag or tool to fill the center of each cupcake and to top each. Top with shaved chocolate if desired. Regarding nutrition, all information includes frosting.

Nutrition:

- Calories: 303

- Fat: 22.1g

- Carbs: 23.5g

- Protein: 8.2g

Chapter 15.

Diabetic Smoothies and Ice

Creams Recipes

40. Green Smoothie

Preparation Time: 12 Minutes

Cooking Time: 0 Minutes

Servings: 2

Ingredients:

- 1 cup vanilla almond milk (unsweetened)

- ¼ ripe avocado, chopped

- 1 cup kale, chopped

- 1 banana

- 2 teaspoons honey

- 1 tablespoon chia seeds

- 1 cup ice cubes

Directions:

1. Combine all the ingredients in a blender.

2. Process until creamy.

Nutrition:

Calories: 343

Carbohydrates: 14.7g

Protein: 5.9g

Conclusion

O ne thing you should do is look for a diabetic dessert cookbook that includes your favorite desserts and go from there. Since you are making them yourself, without all the excess sugar and extra calories, this means that you will be able to indulge in some of your favorite sweets without having to worry about being unhealthy.

The best part about diabetic desserts is that they are a great idea if you are trying to lose weight. This is because you can eat them with the rest of your meals instead of by themselves. This means that you will not have to worry about overeating sweets or getting fat from overeating desserts.

Diabetic dessert cookbooks are an excellent idea for people who live an active lifestyle and want to include healthy desserts in their diet plan. This is because they are easy to make, or you could also prepare them ahead of time and freeze them.

This is an excellent idea if you have more than one meal per day, as it allows you to include dessert in all of your meals.

The main benefit of diabetic desserts is that they are high in protein and low in sugar, so they can be used as a substitute for regular vegetables if needed. This is great for people trying to lose weight and need to replace high-calorie, sugary foods with more protein or other healthy alternatives.

We cheer you to snap some photographs of desserts you made with this cookbook and post them on Instagram and Facebook. Please give time to see our new cookbook!

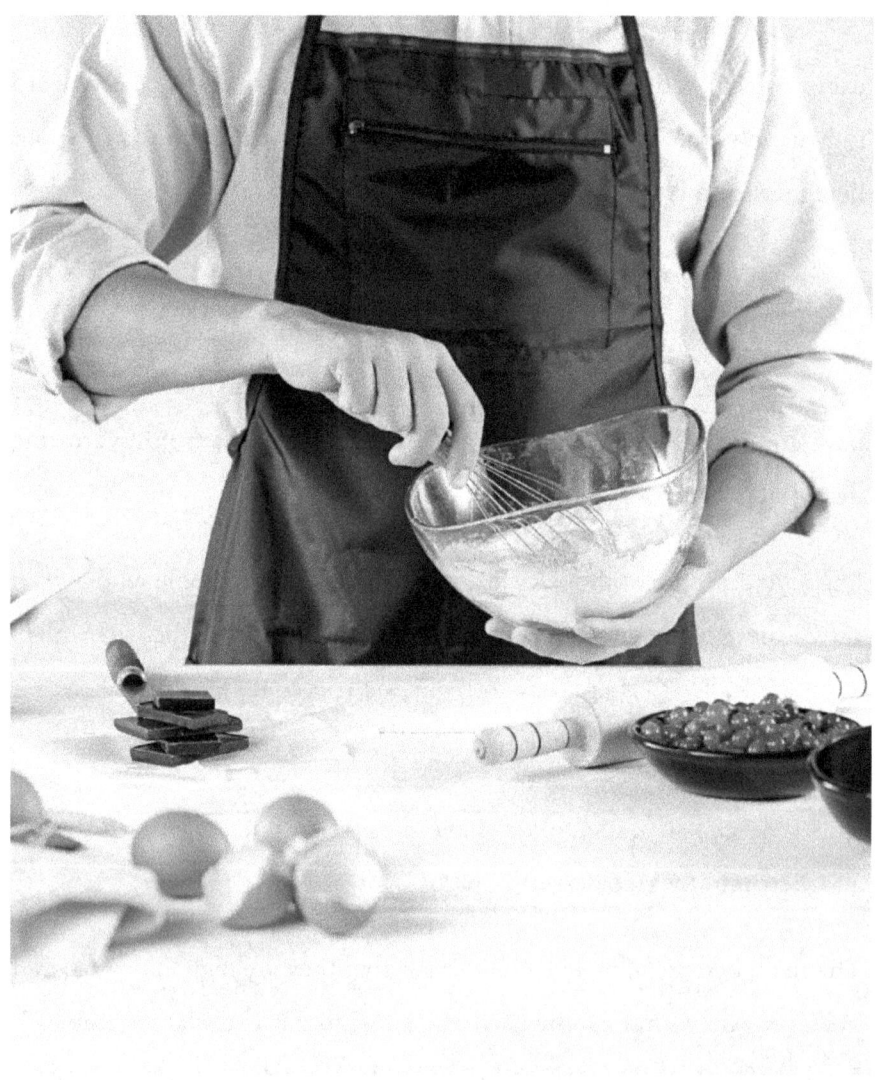

CPSIA information can be obtained
at www.ICGtesting.com
Printed in the USA
BVHW091503140621
609529BV00007B/1976

9 781911 685623